Conscious Care

A Nurse's Guide to Mindful Health

By

Taylor Rose

Legal & Disclaimer

The information in this book is not designed to replace or take the place of any form of medical or professional advice. It is not meant to replace the need for independent medical, financial, legal, or other professional advice or services as may be required. The content and information in this book have been provided for educational and entertainment purposes only.

The content and information contained in this book have been compiled from sources deemed reliable, and it is accurate to the best of the author's knowledge, information, and belief. However, the author cannot guarantee its accuracy and validity and cannot be held liable for any errors and omissions. Further, changes are periodically made to this book as and when needed. Where appropriate and necessary, you must consult a professional (including but not limited to your doctor, attorney, financial advisor, or such other professional advisor) before using any of the suggested remedies, techniques, or information in this book.

Upon using the contents and information contained in this book, you agree to hold harmless the author from and against any damages, costs, and expenses, including any legal fees potentially resulting from the application of any of the information provided by this book. This disclaimer applies to any loss, damages, or injury caused by the use and application, whether directly or indirectly, of any advice or information presented, whether for breach of contract, tort, negligence, personal injury, criminal intent, or under any other cause of action.

You agree to accept all risks of using the information presented in this book.

You agree that by continuing to read this book, where appropriate and necessary, you shall consult a professional (including but not limited to your doctor, attorney, financial advisor, or such other advisor as needed) before using any of the suggested remedies, techniques, or information in this book.

Table Of Contents

THIS BOOK IS DEDICATED TO YOU

To all the caregivers, nurturers, lovers, and dreamers, this book is dedicated to you. Whether you identify as a woman, man, mother, father, grandmother, grandfather, aunt, or uncle, you carry countless responsibilities and wear many hats. Each role serves its purpose, bringing both challenges and rewards while leaving little room for your own well-being and conscious living.

"From a Nurse's Guide to Mindful health" is penned for those who have experienced profound exhaustion, not merely physical but mental and emotional. This book is a tribute to those who awaken each day feeling trapped in the cycle of their lives, echoing Tupac Shakur's infamous words, "That's just the way it is." It speaks to those who, despite their dreams and ambitions, remain confined within the boundaries of their comfort zones due to fear of the unknown. It's for those battling chronic illnesses, enduring unrelenting pain amidst life's relentless pace, and for those clinging to the faintest glimmer of hope that things will eventually be okay, that they will somehow make it through.

Know that you are not alone on this journey. These pages will explore the profound connection between mental and physical health.

Conscious Care

I've penned this book to guide and support others on their journeys. Drawing from my struggles as a nurse, mother, daughter, and human being, I aim to bridge the gap between our emotional well-being and holistic healing process. Years ago, my life was consumed by depression, chronic stress, toxic relationships, and a pervasive pessimism that tainted both my home and work life. Each morning brought a sense of existential dread, questioning how I ended up in such a place. Negative self-talk plagued my thoughts, leaving me drained and doubting my worth. Sleepless nights and stress-induced headaches became my norm.

Everything changed in the summer of 2021. I realized that my problems weren't just affecting me but were casting a shadow over my children's lives as well. I knew I had to seek help, not just for myself, but for them. Therapy provided some relief, but it wasn't until I delved into the power of my thoughts and beliefs that I truly began to heal. Through journaling, meditation, and affirmations, I gradually shifted my mindset. My headaches lessened, my sleep returned, and I regained my focus at work. This transformation underscored the profound impact of proactive mental health strategies on both personal and professional success. As a registered nurse, I've witnessed firsthand how our mental and emotional states influence our physical well-being and healing processes. This journey is an invitation to transform your understanding of health and wellness. "The Conscious Caregiver: A Nurse's Guide to Mental Health" is more than just a book; it's a revelation. Within its pages, we illuminate the symbiotic relationship between mind and body, offering practical strategies to enhance your overall well-being.

Why this book matters

This book will be your light, showing you the way to a happier and more fulfilling life. I aim to empower individuals to unlock the innate healing potential residing within each of us by delving into the realms of mindfulness and conscious living. Central to our exploration is the intricate interplay between mental, emotional, and physical well-being—a concept encapsulated by the profound notion of the "mind-body connection" within healthcare. According to this principle, our emotional and psychological states wield considerable influence over our physical health. Negative emotions and stress, for instance, can compromise our immune system and exacerbate physical ailments, while cultivating optimism and emotional resilience can foster healing and bolster overall well-being.

Objectives

By the end of this book, you will

- Physically gain profound insights into reshaping subconscious beliefs to nurture health and vitality.

- Learn effective techniques for reprogramming your subconscious mind to optimize health outcomes.

- Acquire practical strategies for cultivating a positive mindset, thus fortifying overall health and resilience.

- Understand the symbiotic relationship between positive thinking and mental well-being, leading to tangible health benefits.

How to use this book as a compass on your journey

- **Reflection Questions:** Engage deeply with the material by pondering thought-provoking queries.

- **Inspirational Quotes:** Draw inspiration from timeless wisdom to invigorate your journey.

- **Assessment:** Evaluate your progress and insights gained along the way.

- **Affirmations:** Harness the power of positive affirmations to reinforce newfound perspectives and intentions.

- **Gratitude Prompts:** Cultivate an attitude of gratitude to enrich your daily life and well-being.

- **Action Plan:** Craft a personalized roadmap aligned with the principles outlined in this book, guiding you towards transformative growth and holistic well-being.

INTRODUCTION

"The Conscious Care: A Nurse's Guide to Mindful Health" is a journey into the profound significance of mindfulness and heightened awareness in fostering optimal health. Through this exploration, the book sets out to achieve the following objectives:

- **Raising Awareness:** Have you ever paused to ponder the intricate link between our mental and physical well-being? It's a facet often overlooked but brimming with profound implications. Together, we'll delve into this oft-neglected yet consequential relationship.

- **Providing Knowledge:** With a foundation built on thorough research and evidence, this book offers comprehensive insights into the principles of mindful living. Expect to encounter practical wisdom grounded in scientific understanding.

- **Empowerment:** It is my sincere desire to ignite a sense of empowerment within you—to catalyze proactive efforts toward enhancing your health, resilience, and overall quality of life. Through knowledge and understanding, we unlock the potential for transformative self-care.

- **Inspiring Action:** Beyond mere comprehension lies the call to action. I aim to stir within you a commitment to infuse mindfulness and conscious living into your daily existence. By cultivating these practices, we pave the path toward a life imbued with vitality and fulfillment.

- **Bridging the Divide:** As we navigate the intricate terrain of the mind-body relationship, let us endeavor to bridge the chasm between these realms. Together, we envision a future characterized by a holistic approach to health and wellness—one that recognizes and honors the profound interconnectedness of mind, body, and spirit.

Embark on this journey with me as we uncover the secrets to conscious health and well-being. Let us unite in our pursuit of a future where care is not merely an act of conscientiousness but a testament to our reverence for the intricate dance between mind, body, and spirit.

Chapter 1: Understanding The Relationship Between The Mind And Body

> **The Intricacies of the Mind-Body Connection**

The mind-body connection is a captivating concept that delves into the profound interplay between our mental and emotional states and our physical health. Our thoughts, emotions, and beliefs wield remarkable influence over our bodies, impacting everything from our immune system to our metabolic functions. Negative emotions such as stress, anxiety, and depression can manifest as tangible physical symptoms, while positive emotions like joy and optimism can bolster our overall well-being. Cultivating a positive mindset and nurturing our emotional health can not only enhance our physical health but also enrich our lives immeasurably.

> **The Bidirectional Relationship Between Physical and Emotional Well-Being**

Did you know that our physical health significantly impacts our emotional and psychological well-being and vice versa? Indeed, the intricate interplay between these dimensions is undeniable. Therefore, it's crucial to prioritize the care of both our physical and emotional health, recognizing their interconnected nature as vital components of our overall well-being.

➤ Ancient Wisdom and Modern Insights: Perspectives on Mind-Body Healing

Throughout history, diverse civilizations and cultures have recognized the profound implications of the mind-body connection, shaping their healing practices accordingly. Ancient healing traditions from India, China, Greece, and Egypt acknowledged the inseparable link between mental, physical, and spiritual health. For instance, Ayurveda, an ancient Indian healing system, emphasized holistic well-being by addressing the entirety of the individual, not merely their physical ailments.

Similarly, Traditional Chinese Medicine (TCM) sought to restore balance to the body's energy, known as qi, through practices such as acupuncture and herbal medicine. Even the ancient Greek philosopher Hippocrates advocated for a holistic approach to healthcare, emphasizing the importance of understanding the person behind the illness.

➤ Integrating Ancient Wisdom with Modern Science

Contemporary pioneers in psychology, such as Sigmund Freud and Carl Jung, further explored the intricate relationship between psychological and physical wellness. Their groundbreaking work paved the way for integrative medicine, which combines conventional medical practices with complementary and alternative therapies to treat the whole person.

By synthesizing the insights gleaned from ancient traditions with the findings of contemporary research, we continue to deepen our understanding of the mind-body connection and its profound implications for health and healing.

Scientific Insights: Unveiling the Impact of Mental States on Physical Well-Being

Recent scientific studies have provided compelling evidence of the profound impact of mental states on physical health:

➢ The Placebo and Nocebo Effects

Research by Benedetti et al. (2015) underscores the profound influence of belief and anticipation on health outcomes. The placebo effect, for instance, activates neurotransmitters and brain regions associated with pain relief. Conversely, the nocebo effect, as observed by Colloca and Miller (2011), highlights how negative expectations can exacerbate symptoms and diminish treatment efficacy. Recognizing the pivotal role of mindset in symptom severity and treatment outcomes is imperative in addressing health concerns effectively.

➢ Stress and Immune Function

Chronic mental and emotional stress has been linked to compromised immune function and overall health. Studies by Cohen et al. (2012) reveal the detrimental impact of cognitive and emotional stressors on immune response. Additionally, research by Kiecolt-Glaser et al. (2015) demonstrates how stress-induced inflammation exacerbates chronic conditions like diabetes and cardiovascular disease. Understanding the intricate interplay between stress and immune function is paramount in promoting holistic well-being.

➢ Mindfulness and Pain Management

Evidence suggests that mindfulness-based therapies offer promising avenues for alleviating chronic pain. Studies by Zeidan et al. (2011) and Garland et al. (2014) illustrate how mindfulness practices can modulate brain activity and processing systems, thereby mitigating pain perception and discomfort. By embracing mindfulness, individuals can cultivate a newfound relationship with pain, fostering resilience and well-being.

➢ Optimism and Heart Health

Optimism emerges as a potent determinant of heart health outcomes, as evidenced by research conducted by Boehm et al. (2012). Optimistic individuals exhibit superior cardiovascular health and a reduced risk of developing cardiovascular disease compared to their pessimistic counterparts. Further studies by Giltay et al. (2006) and Tindle et al. (2009) highlight the multifaceted benefits of optimism, including healthier lifestyle choices, reduced inflammation, and enhanced cardiovascular functioning.

➢ Psychosocial Factors and Cancer Survival

The psychosocial landscape profoundly influences cancer patients' treatment outcomes and quality of life. Research by Pinquart and Duberstein (2010) and Chida et al. (2008) emphasizes the pivotal role of social support and coping mechanisms in fostering positive treatment experiences and overall survival rates. By harnessing the mind-body connection, patients can optimize their well-being, mitigate treatment-related complications, and enhance their chances of successful treatment outcomes.

Chapter 2: The Power Of Positive Thinking

> ### The Power of Positive Thinking

Positive thinking entails adopting an optimistic and constructive outlook on life. It involves directing our focus towards the positive aspects of situations rather than dwelling on the negative. Positive thinkers view setbacks as opportunities for growth and learning rather than insurmountable obstacles.

However, positive thinking doesn't entail ignoring or denying reality; rather, it involves reframing our perspective to see challenges in a more positive light. This includes maintaining a hopeful attitude toward the future, appreciating the present moment, and nurturing confidence in our abilities. By cultivating a positive mindset, individuals are better equipped to overcome obstacles and achieve their goals.

> ### Benefits of Positive Thinking on Well-being

Fostering an optimistic mindset can profoundly impact overall well-being. By focusing on the positive aspects of life, individuals can reduce stress levels, enhance resilience in the face of challenges, elevate mood, and experience greater happiness. Moreover, scientific studies have demonstrated that optimism correlates with improved immune function, faster recovery from injuries and illnesses, and a reduced risk of developing chronic diseases.

➤ How Optimism Affects Health

Scientific research underscores the significant impact of positive thinking on health and healing:

- Positive thinking bolsters the body's immune response, leading to more robust defenses against infections and diseases (Segerstrom & Sephton, 2010).

- Optimistic individuals tend to experience quicker recovery rates after surgery or injury compared to their pessimistic counterparts (Rasmussen et al., 2009). Furthermore,

- Optimism is associated with better health outcomes and lower mortality rates across various health conditions (Chida et al., 2008).

- Optimism is linked to improved heart health, with optimistic individuals exhibiting a reduced risk of developing cardiovascular disease (Boehm et al., 2012).

- Positive thinking can help manage pain and its symptoms by increasing the production of endorphins, the body's natural painkillers (Edwards et al., 2006). Additionally, optimism contributes to psychological well-being and resilience, aiding in coping with chronic pain (Zautra et al., 2005).

- Optimism reduces anxiety, depression, and psychological distress, promoting greater happiness and life satisfaction (Seligman et al., 2006; Tugade et al., 2004).

> ## Conclusion and Practical Tips

In conclusion, cultivating a positive attitude is a powerful tool for improving mental and physical health, enhancing energy levels, resilience, and overall quality of life. Developing a positive outlook requires continuous effort and the cultivation of habits promoting optimism and resilience.

Inspiring individuals like Michael J. Fox, Magic Johnson, Robin Roberts, and Demi Lovato serve as shining examples of the transformative power of positive thinking and self-care. By adopting gratitude practices, challenging negative thoughts, surrounding ourselves with positive influences, and nurturing supportive relationships, we can shift our perspective on life and navigate challenges with greater ease.

Remember, a positive outlook can make all the difference in how we experience life's ups and downs.

> ## Cultivate Mindfulness Practices

Incorporate mindfulness into your daily routine to cultivate presence and self-acceptance. Through practices such as mindfulness meditation, deep breathing exercises, and body scans, you can develop the capacity to remain calm and composed in any circumstance.

> ## Establish Realistic Goals

Set attainable objectives and celebrate your progress at each milestone. Direct your focus towards what you can influence, and break larger aspirations into smaller, more manageable tasks. Prioritize activities that promote self-care, nurturing your mental, physical, and emotional well-being to sustain a positive mindset.

➢ Prioritize Self-Care

Commit to self-care rituals that encompass physical exercise, nourishing nutrition, sufficient rest, indulging in enjoyable hobbies, and connecting with nature. By tending to your holistic well-being—physically, mentally, and spiritually—you pave the way for a rich and fulfilling life.

Chapter 3: Anxiety And Stress Management

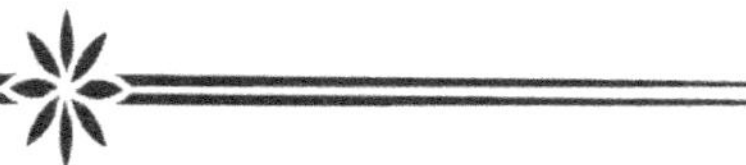

> **Understanding the Impact of Prolonged Stress and Worry**

It is imperative to recognize the profound and wide-ranging effects that prolonged stress and worry can exert on both our physical and emotional well-being. These detrimental consequences encompass various facets, including:

> **Cardiovascular Issues**

Persistent anxiety and stress can impose significant strain on the cardiovascular system. The body's response to stress triggers an elevation in blood pressure, heart rate, and stress hormone levels, such as adrenaline and cortisol. Over time, these physiological changes can exacerbate preexisting cardiovascular conditions such as hypertension, coronary artery disease, and stroke.

> **Weakened Immune System**

Chronic stress compromises immune function, rendering individuals more susceptible to illnesses, infections, and autoimmune disorders. Stress hormones suppress immune cell activity, impairing the body's ability to fend off pathogens and recover effectively.

> **Digestive Problems**

The harmful impact of stress and anxiety extends to the digestive system, precipitating a spectrum of issues ranging from dyspepsia and nausea to indigestion and abdominal discomfort. For individuals grappling with gastrointestinal disorders like peptic ulcers, inflammatory bowel disease (IBD), and irritable bowel syndrome (IBS), chronic stress exacerbates symptoms and significantly diminishes their quality of life.

➤ Musculoskeletal Problems

Stress and anxiety manifest physically, manifesting as muscle tension and stiffness, culminating in ailments such as tension headaches, temporomandibular joint (TMJ) disorder, and fibromyalgia. Suboptimal posture and muscle strain further exacerbate pain and heighten susceptibility to injury.

➤ Mental Health Disorders

Prolonged stress and worry precipitate the onset of mental health disorders, encompassing conditions like post-traumatic stress disorder (PTSD), major depressive disorder, and anxiety disorders. This can precipitate emotional exhaustion, burnout, and a pervasive sense of diminished well-being.

➤ Cognitive Impairment

Chronic stress takes a toll on cognitive function, manifesting as difficulties in concentration, decision-making, and memory retention.

➤ Disruptions to Sleep

Chronic stress disrupts sleep patterns, leading to insomnia and poor sleep quality, further exacerbating the cycle of stress and its associated health consequences.

By integrating mindfulness practices and stress-management techniques into their daily routines, individuals can bolster their resilience, enhance their overall health, and achieve a more harmonious balance in life.

Relaxation and Stress Reduction Practices Based on Mindfulness

In today's fast-paced society, stress and anxiety have become pervasive, impacting both mental and physical well-being. Fortunately, numerous mindfulness-based relaxation practices can help alleviate stress and foster inner peace. Mindfulness involves being fully present in the moment and acknowledging one's internal experiences without judgment, encompassing emotions, body sensations, and thoughts.

One highly effective approach to managing stress is through mindfulness-based relaxation techniques, such as yoga, tai chi, body scans, deep breathing, and meditation. These practices facilitate a deeper understanding of oneself, aid in emotional regulation, and enhance inner strength and balance by fostering awareness of the body, thoughts, and feelings.

Yoga integrates physical postures, breathing techniques, and meditation to promote relaxation, flexibility, and strength. Similarly, tai chi, a Chinese martial art, incorporates gentle movements, deep breathing, and meditation to reduce stress and enhance balance. Body scans involve directing attention to different body parts, noticing physical sensations, and releasing tension to induce relaxation. Deep breathing exercises entail slow, deliberate breaths to calm both mind and body. Meditation entails quieting the mind and focusing on the present moment, effectively reducing stress and fostering inner peace.

Incorporating mindfulness into daily routines can significantly reduce stress levels and promote relaxation in both body and mind. Consistent practice of mindfulness-based approaches equips individuals with the tools to navigate life's challenges gracefully and cultivate a healthier relationship with oneself and the world. Ultimately, mindfulness empowers individuals to lead happier, healthier lives by enhancing self-awareness and fostering resilience in the face of life's complexities.

Activities to Do Each Day to Make Stress Management a Part of Your Routine

To foster health and resilience amidst life's challenges, it's crucial to integrate stress management techniques into your daily routine. Here are some exercises and activities to help you incorporate mindfulness-based practices into your everyday life:

- **Mindful Breathing:** Set aside time each day to practice mindful breathing. Find a comfortable position, close your eyes, and focus on your breath. Allow the sensations of each inhale and exhale to guide you into a calm and present state.

- **Body Scan Meditation:** Start at the base of your skull and gradually relax your entire body as you scan down. Notice any tension or discomfort and visualize releasing stress with each breath.

- **Mindful Walking:** Take a stroll outdoors, tuning into the present moment and engaging all your senses. Feel the ground beneath your feet, listen to the rustling of leaves, and bask in the warmth of the sun. Let go of worries and distractions, fully immersing yourself in the experience.

- . **Keeping a Gratitude Journal:** Dedicate a few minutes each day to write down three things you're grateful for. Cultivate feelings of gratitude and abundance as you reflect on the positive aspects of your life, no matter how small.

- **Mindful Eating:** Practice mindful eating by savoring each bite and focusing on the flavors, textures, and sensations in your mouth. Appreciate how your body feels as you nourish it with food.

- **Progressive Muscle Relaxation:** Learn to release tension and alleviate stress through progressive muscle relaxation. Tense and then gradually release each muscle group from your toes to your head, promoting deep relaxation.

- **Picture Yourself in a Calm Environment:** Utilize guided imagery or visualization techniques to transport yourself to a calm and tranquil environment. Close your eyes and immerse yourself in the sensory details of this imaginary sanctuary, allowing a sense of peace to wash over you.

Incorporating these mindfulness practices into your daily life can enhance your self-awareness, resilience, and overall well-being. By cultivating these habits, you'll be better equipped to manage stress and achieve a healthier balance in life.

Chapter 4: What Subconscious Beliefs And Thought Patterns Affect Your Health

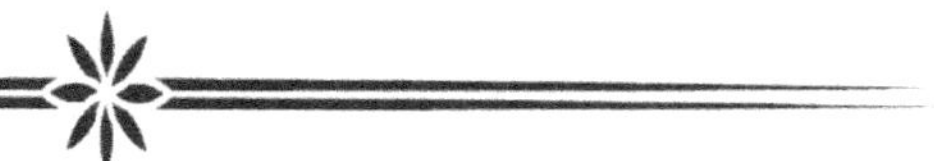

Our beliefs and thought patterns wield significant influence over our well-being. Both research studies and real-life examples underscore how even subconscious beliefs can profoundly shape our health behaviors. Let's delve deeper into these examples:

- **Self-image and Identity**: Our beliefs regarding our abilities and self-worth profoundly impact our health behaviors. Individuals with low self-esteem may avoid seeking medical assistance or neglect self-care practices.

- **Expectations and Mindset**: Our mindset plays a pivotal role in determining our health outcomes. Those harboring positive expectations about their capacity to enhance their health are more inclined to adopt healthy behaviors and reap positive results.

- **Emotional Coping Mechanisms**: Subconscious beliefs mold our emotional coping mechanisms and subsequent health behaviors. Instances of resorting to unhealthy coping mechanisms like smoking or overeating during times of stress highlight the profound influence of ingrained beliefs on our actions.

- **Social and Cultural Influences:** Social and cultural norms significantly shape our health beliefs. Individuals may unwittingly adopt unhealthy behaviors modeled by family members or influenced by societal norms, disregarding their detrimental effects on health.

- **Automatic Decision-Making:** Our subconscious beliefs and thought patterns often drive automatic behaviors, sometimes conflicting with our health objectives. Making impulsive food choices or skipping exercise without conscious consideration of the consequences exemplify this phenomenon.

- **Limiting Beliefs and Self-Sabotage:** Beliefs regarding our capacity to effect change in our health can precipitate self-sabotaging actions that undermine efforts to adopt healthier habits. Recognizing how our beliefs influence our actions is crucial in overcoming self-imposed limitations.

Guidance on Identifying and Challenging Limiting Beliefs:

Identifying and challenging limiting beliefs is pivotal for fostering personal growth and well-being. These beliefs, which are negative thoughts and perceptions, hinder us from leading fulfilling lives. Employ the following strategies to identify and challenge these limiting beliefs:

- **Self-Reflection:** Engage in self-reflection to pinpoint limiting beliefs. Observe your thoughts, beliefs, and behaviors, noting any recurring patterns hindering your progress or causing distress. Journaling can aid in exploring your inner thoughts and uncovering underlying beliefs.

- **Pay Attention to Negative Self-Talk:** Negative self-talk often indicates the presence of limiting beliefs. Pay attention to your internal dialogue. Are you excessively critical or harsh? Challenge negative self-talk by questioning its validity. Assess if there is evidence supporting these beliefs or if they are rooted in assumptions or past experiences.

- **Examine Triggers:** Triggers, whether they be situations or events, often provoke strong emotional reactions or self-doubt. They can serve as valuable indicators of underlying limiting beliefs. By identifying these triggers, you empower yourself to reframe your thoughts and responses in such situations.

- **Seek Feedback:** Reaching out to trusted friends, family members, or a therapist for feedback can prove instrumental in identifying and challenging limiting beliefs. External perspectives can shed light on our beliefs and aid in challenging distorted thinking patterns.

- **Question Assumptions:** Challenge assumptions and beliefs that may impede your progress by evaluating their relevance to your current circumstances. Ask yourself whether these beliefs are beneficial or if they are outdated and no longer applicable to your present situation.

Tools for Reframing Negative Self-Talk and Promoting Self-Compassion

Once you've identified limiting beliefs, utilize these tools to reframe negative self-talk and nurture self-compassion:

Cognitive Restructuring: Challenge and reframe negative thoughts using cognitive restructuring techniques. Replace self-critical statements with more realistic and compassionate alternatives. For instance, instead of saying, "I'm a failure," reframe it as, "I made a mistake, but it doesn't define my worth as a person."

Positive Affirmations: Counteract negative self-talk with positive affirmations that reinforce self-belief. Craft affirmations reflecting your strengths, values, and aspirations, and repeat them regularly to internalize positive messages about yourself.

Mindfulness and Self-Compassion Practices: Cultivate a compassionate attitude toward yourself through mindfulness and self-compassion practices. Extend the same kindness and understanding to yourself that you would offer to a friend facing similar challenges.

Gratitude Practice: Foster gratitude by focusing on the positive aspects of your life and acknowledging your strengths and accomplishments. Maintain a gratitude journal and jot down three things you're thankful for each day, regardless of their size.

Seek Support: Reach out to supportive friends, family members, or a therapist for encouragement and validation. Surround yourself with individuals who uplift and empower you, and don't hesitate to seek assistance when needed.

> **Discover your "sanctuary!"**

Everyone has that special activity that uplifts their spirit, calms their soul, and serves as an oasis of tranquility during tough moments. For me, that special something is music. Regardless of the trials I face, music has a way of making my soul sing, bringing peace and tranquility. Whether it's a sleepless night or overwhelming stress, music has the power to elevate my energy and change my entire mood. Whether it's during quiet car rides, enjoying scenic views, or listening to the rhythm of waves crashing against the shore, music and the sound of the sea bring me profound peace and joy.

Discovering and embracing your source of solace and joy isn't just a hobby; it's an essential tool for weathering life's most brutal storms. It provides solace and peace precisely when you need it most. By actively challenging limiting beliefs, reframing negative self-talk, and fostering self-compassion, you can cultivate a more positive and empowering mindset that supports your overall well-being and personal growth. Remember, this process requires time and effort, but the results are undoubtedly worth it.

Chapter 5: Nurturing Resilience And Emotional Well-Being

Resilience is a multifaceted concept that refers to an individual's capacity to navigate challenging situations and stress by cultivating strength, adaptability, and effective coping mechanisms. It encompasses emotional regulation, problem-solving abilities, and a sense of purpose that enables individuals to thrive amidst adversity. Unlike innate traits, resilience is something that can be nurtured and reinforced over time through a variety of life experiences.

During times of adversity, resilience plays a pivotal role in maintaining health and well-being in several key ways:

- **Emotional Well-being:** Resilient individuals demonstrate greater emotional resilience, allowing them to manage their emotions more effectively during difficult circumstances. This emotional stability fosters a sense of confidence and optimism, contributing to overall mental health.

- **Coping with Stress:** Resilience equips individuals with effective coping mechanisms, reducing the negative impact of stress on their physical health. Resilient individuals are less prone to conditions such as high blood pressure, weakened immune systems, and mental health disorders stemming from chronic stress.

- **Adaptability and Flexibility:** Resilience cultivates adaptability and flexibility, enabling individuals to navigate obstacles and devise creative solutions. This proactive approach empowers individuals to take charge of their health and seek support and resources when needed.

- **Problem-Solving Skills:** Resilient individuals possess strong problem-solving abilities and resourcefulness, allowing them to overcome challenges effectively.

- **Sense of Purpose and Meaning:** Resilient individuals often derive a sense of purpose and meaning from their experiences, providing them with motivation and resilience during difficult times. This intrinsic drive serves as a guiding force, helping individuals maintain their health and well-being.

- **Social Support and Connection:** Resilient individuals benefit from strong support networks and healthy relationships, enabling them to seek assistance when necessary and cope with stress more effectively.

Resilience serves as a protective factor against the adverse effects of stress on health. By developing resilience through effective coping strategies, emotional regulation, problem-solving skills, and social support, individuals can maintain their health and well-being even amidst challenging circumstances.

Strategies for Enhancing Emotional Well-Being and Coping Skills

Enhancing emotional well-being and coping skills is crucial for leading a fulfilling life, especially in the face of life's challenges. Here are ten detailed strategies to promote emotional well-being and cultivate practical coping skills:

- **Practice Mindfulness:** Engage in mindfulness activities like meditation, deep breathing, and body scans to observe your thoughts and emotions without judgment, enhancing clarity and composure in challenging situations.

- **Develop Emotional Awareness:** Recognize, understand, and manage your emotions by acknowledging their validity and exploring them through journaling, self-reflection, and expressive arts.

- **Build a Strong Support Network:** Cultivate meaningful connections with supportive individuals who offer empathy, perspective, and practical assistance during difficult times.

- **Practice Self-Compassion:** Treat yourself with kindness and understanding, offering the same warmth and care you would extend to a friend facing similar challenges.

- **Develop Problem-Solving Skills:** Break down problems into manageable steps, brainstorm solutions, and focus on constructive actions rather than dwelling on obstacles.

- **Seek Professional Help:** Don't hesitate to reach out to a mental health professional or counselor for valuable support, tools, and strategies.

- **Engage in Healthy Lifestyle Habits:** Prioritize self-care activities such as exercise, nutritious eating, sleep, and relaxation techniques to support physical and mental well-being.

- **Set and Prioritize Self-Care:** Establish boundaries, learn to avoid draining commitments, and prioritize activities that replenish and rejuvenate you.

- **Practice Gratitude and Positivity:** Cultivate gratitude and adopt a positive mindset by reframing negative thoughts, fostering resilience and optimism.

- **Engage in Relaxation Techniques:** Incorporate progressive muscle relaxation, guided imagery, or aromatherapy into your routine to reduce stress and promote relaxation.

By integrating these strategies into your life, you can enhance emotional well-being, develop coping skills, and build resilience to navigate life's challenges confidently.

Conclusion

"The Conscious Care: A Nurse's Guide to Mindful Health" is an empowering resource that emphasizes the profound impact of mindset on overall health. Through exploring the mind-body connection, historical perspectives, scientific research, and real-life examples, this book equips readers with the tools to transform health behaviors by reshaping thoughts and beliefs. By addressing the negative effects of anxiety and stress and promoting positive thinking, the book guides readers in cultivating mental wellness, mindfulness, and resilience. Additionally, it underscores the importance of self-care for healthcare providers and caregivers, which is essential for delivering compassionate care and fostering meaningful relationships with patients and families. "Conscious Care" serves as a comprehensive guide to mindful living and compassionate caregiving, encouraging readers to embark on a journey towards wellness and personal growth while also empowering them to support others in their care. "Take a deep breath and whisper to yourself, 'I got this!'".

Affirmations

1. I am in control of my thoughts and my health.

2. I lead my life with positivity and purpose every day.

3. I hold the power to transform my health through my thoughts.

4. My mind and body are in perfect harmony.

5. I am resilient, strong, and capable of overcoming challenges.

6. Peace and relaxation flow through me with every breath I take.

7. I deserve a stress-free and joyful life.

8. Each day, I grow more confident in the power of my positive thoughts.

9. I release all fears and embrace new growth opportunities.

10. My body heals as I fill my mind with positive thoughts.

11. I am patient with myself and accept that good health is a journey.

12. I am learning to manage stress effectively every day.

13. Every challenge is an opportunity to improve my emotional and physical well-being.

14. I am kind to myself and speak positively about my body and mind.

15. My emotional resilience is growing stronger each day.

16. I trust in my ability to nurture my mind and body.

17. I am dedicated to discovering deep peace through mindfulness.

18. My health journey is guided by love and self-compassion.

19. I am committed to breaking free from limiting beliefs that hinder my health.

20. I celebrate each victory on my path to well-being, no matter how small.

Adopt a mindset that promotes holistic health and resilience.

Reflection Questions

1. What are the main sources of stress in my life, and how do they affect my physical health?

2. How do I typically respond to stress, and what can I change about my response to improve my well-being?

3. How can I incorporate more positive thinking into my daily routine?

4. How do my thoughts influence my physical symptoms or health conditions?

5. What are some limiting beliefs I hold about my health or abilities, and where did they come from?

6. How can I challenge and reframe these limiting beliefs to support my health and goals?

7. What relaxation techniques have I tried, and which ones have been the most effective for me?

8. How do I currently manage anxiety and stress, and what new methods can I like to try?

9. What does resilience mean to me personally, and how have I demonstrated resilience in my life?

10. How can I nurture my emotional well-being daily?

11. How can I practice self-compassion when I'm feeling down or critical of myself?

12. What have I learned about the mind-body connection that was new to me?

13. How can I use this book as a compass to guide my journey toward better health?

14. Reflecting on a time when positive thinking significantly impacted a challenging situation in my life. What happened?

15. What subconscious beliefs about health am I aware of that could be impacting my well-being?

16. How do I feel after participating in mindfulness or relaxation practices?

17. What daily activities can I introduce into my life to help manage stress more effectively?

18. In what ways have I allowed fear of the unknown to limit my actions, and how can I overcome this?

19. How has my perspective on health and wellness changed after reading this book?

20. What are my main takeaways from "Conscious Care," and how can I apply them to my life?

The questions are designed to expand your thinking about the concepts discussed in the book and encourage personal growth and self-awareness concerning mental, emotional, and physical health.

30-Day Action Plan

Day 1: Self-Assessment

- **Activity**: Write down your health status, emotions, and any stressors affecting you.

Day 2: Set Clear Goals

- **Activity**: Define specific, measurable goals for your mental and physical health for the next 30 days.

Day 3: Introduction to Mindfulness

- **Activity**: Read about mindfulness and practice a 5-minute meditation.

Day 4: Positive Affirmations

- **Activity**: Create a list of personal affirmations based on your goals from Day 2.

Day 5: Identifying Stressors

- **Activity**: Journal about the main sources of stress in your life.

Day 6: Learning Relaxation Techniques

- **Activity**: Try a new relaxation technique, such as deep breathing or progressive muscle relaxation.

Day 7: Reflection

- **Activity**: Reflect on the week and journal about any changes in your stress and anxiety levels.

Day 8: Introduction to Positive Thinking

- **Activity**: Read a chapter on the power of positive thinking and note the key takeaways.

Day 9: Applying Positive Thinking

- **Activity**: Replace a negative thought with a positive one throughout the day.

Day 10: Explore Physical Activity

- **Activity**: Engage in 30 minutes of physical activity you enjoy.

Day 11: Mind-Body Connection

- **Activity**: Write about how your body reacted to the positive changes in thought and activity.

Day 12: Stress Management Techniques

- **Activity**: Learn and apply a new stress management strategy.

Day 13: Tackling Limiting Beliefs

- **Activity**: Identify and write down one limiting belief and challenge it.

Day 14: Mid-Point Reflection

- **Activity**: Review your goals and progress and adjust your plan.

Day 15: Emotional Well-Being Strategies

- **Activity**: Practice self-compassion with a specific self-care activity.

Day 16: Cultivating Resilience

- **Activity**: Read about resilience and write in a journal about a time you demonstrated resilience.

Day 17: Daily Routine Adjustment

- **Activity**: Incorporate one positive habit into your daily routine.

Day 18: Enhancing Coping Skills

- **Activity**: Try a coping strategy for handling emotional distress.

Day 19: Connection and Support

- **Activity**: Reach out to a friend or support group to share experiences and gain insights.

Day 20: Dive Deeper into Mindfulness

- **Activity**: Attend a mindfulness class or follow an online guided meditation.

Day 21: Weekly Reflection

- **Activity**: Reflect on your mindfulness journey and its impacts.

Day 22: Revisit Goals

- **Activity**: Ensure your goals align with your learning and experiences.

Day 23: Positive Environmental Changes

Conscious Care

- **Activity**: Modify your living space to reduce stress and enhance positivity.

Day 24: Advanced Positive Affirmations

- **Activity**: Review and revise your affirmations list based on your current mindset.

Day 25: Mindfulness in Daily Activities

- **Activity**: Practice being mindful during routine activities like eating or walking.

Day 26: Exploring Subconscious Beliefs

- **Activity**: Delve deeper into one subconscious belief that affects your health.

Day 27: Implementing a New Hobby

- **Activity**: Start a new hobby that improves your mental health (e.g., painting, writing).

Day 28: Self-Evaluation

- **Activity**: Evaluate your mental, emotional, and physical health changes.

Day 29: Plan for Continuing Growth

- **Activity**: Develop a plan for continuing the practices you've learned after the 30 days.

Day 30: Final Reflection and Celebration

- **Activity**: Reflect on your journey and celebrate your achievements and growth.

NOTE FROM THE AUTHOR

Dear Reader,

As you reflect on this book, know it was written with a deep sense of dedication and care for you. I understand the journey of seeking wellness and balance because I have walked this path filled with challenges, discoveries, and transformative moments.

Throughout this book, I've shared insights and strategies that have been my companions during my times of profound exhaustion and less-than-optimal health. I hope they will guide you, illuminating your path toward a more abundant, joyful, balanced, and healthy life.

You may find some days more challenging than others, and that's perfectly okay. Remember, every step forward, no matter how small is a step towards a greater understanding of the miraculous connection between your mind and body. I encourage you to embrace this journey with an open heart and a curious mind, allowing yourself to explore new ways of thinking and being.

This book is more than just words on paper—it is a token of my commitment to your well-being and a reflection of the invisible bond that connects all of us who strive for better health and happiness.

Take your time with each page, reflect deeply on the questions, and apply the practices that resonate most. You are not alone on this journey; we are together, exploring the vast landscape of human health and emotional resilience.

Thank you for trusting me to be a part of your journey. May these words offer comfort, inspire change, and bring you closer to the peace and health you deserve.

With all my heart,

-- Taylor Rose

REFERENCES

1. Crum, A. J., Salovey, P., & Achor, S. (2013). Rethinking stress: The role of mindsets in determining the stress response. *Journal of Personality and Social Psychology, 104*(4), 716–733.

2. Langer, E. J., & Moldoveanu, M. (2000). The construct of mindfulness. *Journal of Social Issues, 56*(1), 1–9.

3. Kiviniemi, M. T., Ellis, E. M., Hall, M. G., & Moss, J. L. (2018). Association between self-reported emotional self-efficacy and perceived ability to influence health in a community sample: A multiple mediation analysis. *Stress and Health, 34*(4), 473–480.

4. Williams, D. R., & Mohammed, S. A. (2009). Discrimination and racial health disparities: Evidence and needed research. *Journal of Behavioral Medicine, 32*(1), 20–47.

5. Bargh, J. A., & Chartrand, T. L. (1999). The unbearable automaticity of being. *American Psychologist, 54*(7), 462–479.

6. Dweck, C. S. (2008). Mindset: The new psychology of success. Random House.

7. Keng, S. L., Smoski, M. J., & Robins, C. J. (2011). Effects of mindfulness on psychological health: A review of empirical studies. *Clinical Psychology Review, 31*(6), 1041–1056.

8. Shapiro, S. L., Carlson, L. E., Astin, J. A., & Freedman, B. (2006). Mechanisms of mindfulness. *Journal of Clinical Psychology, 62*(3), 373–386.

9. Hofmann, S. G., Sawyer, A. T., Witt, A. A., & Oh, D. (2010). *The effect of mindfulness-based therapy on anxiety and depression: A meta-analytic review. Journal of Consulting and Clinical Psychology, 78(2), 169–183.*

10. Segal, Z. V., Williams, J. M. G., & Teasdale, J. D. (2002). *Mindfulness-based cognitive therapy for depression: A new approach to preventing relapse. Guilford Press.*

11. Kabat-Zinn, J. (2003). *Mindfulness-based interventions in context: Past, present, and future. Clinical Psychology: Science and Practice, 10(2), 144–156.*

12. Fredrickson, B. L., Cohn, M. A., Coffey, K. A., Pek, J., & Finkel, S. M. (2008). *Open hearts build lives: Positive emotions, induced through loving-kindness meditation, build consequential personal resources. Journal of Personality and Social Psychology, 95(5), 1045–1062.*

13. Carver, C. S., & Scheier, M. F. (2014). *Dispositional optimism. Trends in Cognitive Sciences, 18(6), 293–299.*

14. Segerstrom, S. C., & Sephton, S. E. (2010). *Optimistic expectancies and cell-mediated immunity: The role of positive affect. Psychological Science, 21(3), 448–455.*

15. Seligman, M. E. P., Steen, T. A., Park, N., & Peterson, C. (2005). *Positive psychology progress: Empirical validation of interventions. American Psychologist, 60(5), 410–421.*

16. Peterson, C., & Bossio, L. M. (2001). *Optimism and physical well-being. In E. C. Chang (Ed.), Optimism and pessimism: Implications for theory, research, and practice (pp. 127–145). American Psychological Association.*

17. Folkman, S., & Moskowitz, J. T. (2000). Positive affect and the other side of coping. *American Psychologist, 55*(6), 647–654.

18. Boehm, J. K., & Kubzansky, L. D. (2012). The heart's content: The association between positive psychological well-being and cardiovascular health. *Psychological Bulletin, 138*(4), 655–691.

19. Diener, E., & Chan, M. Y. (2011). Happy people live longer: Subjective well-being contributes to health and longevity. *Applied Psychology: Health and Well-Being, 3*(1), 1–43.

20. Ryff, C. D., & Singer, B. (2008). Know thyself and become what you are: A eudaimonic approach to psychological well-being. *Journal of Happiness Studies, 9*(1), 13–39.

"Good Will"

Helping others without expectation of anything in return has been proven to lead to increased happiness and satisfaction in life.

I would love to allow you to experience that same feeling during your reading or listening experience today…

All it takes is a few moments of your time to answer one simple question:

Would you make a difference in the life of someone you've never met—without spending any money or seeking recognition for your goodwill?

If so, I have a small request for you.

If you've found value in your reading or listening experience today, I humbly ask that you take a moment to leave an honest review of this book. It won't cost you anything but 30 seconds of your time—just a few seconds to share your thoughts with others.

Your voice can go a long way in helping someone else find the same inspiration and knowledge that you have.

Are you familiar with leaving a review for an Audible, Kindle, or e-reader book? If so, it's simple:

If you're on Audible: just hit the three dots in the top right of your device, click rate & review, then leave a few sentences about the book along with your star rating.

If you're reading on Kindle or an e-reader, scroll to the book's last page and swipe up—the review should prompt from there.

 If you're on a paperback or any other physical format for this book, you can find the book page on Amazon (or wherever you bought this) and leave your review there.